Unlock Radiant Wellness for Women Over 40.

Restore your gut micro biome, shed weight, Reignite Energy with intermittent fasting, Nutrition, and self-care

Maggie D. Keck

Copyright

TABLE OF CONTENT

INTRODUCTION

INTRODUCTION

The Relationship Between the Stomach and the Body

Women's bodies alter significantly as they get older. Changes in hormone levels, changes in metabolism, and lifestyle changes all influence their general health. One important but frequently disregarded factor in all of these changes is intestinal health.

Trillions of bacteria live in our digestive tract, forming a complex ecosystem known as the gut, sometimes called the second brain. We refer to these microscopic residents—bacteria, viruses, fungi, and more—as the micro biome. These microorganisms are not inert observers; rather, they actively impact our well-being, impacting not only digestion but also immunological response, mood modulation, and even weight control.

Why Gut Health Is Important Beyond 40

1. Metabolism and Control of Weight

Women frequently observe changes in their metabolism as they approach their forties. The once consistent rate of burning calories appears to decrease, and persistent weight gain appears more frequently. What if I told you that this process is significantly influenced by the micro biota in your stomach?

Studies show that an unbalanced gut micro biota might contribute to weight gain and make it harder to lose those excess pounds. There are intestinal bacteria that take more energy from the food we eat, which makes losing weight difficult. On the other hand, a varied and flourishing microbiome promotes a healthy metabolism and aids in weight maintenance.

2. Harmony of Hormones

Hormonal changes brought on by menopause, a normal stage of life, can affect anything from mood swings to bone health. Unexpectedly, these hormonal shifts are influenced by the intestinal microbiota. It takes a role in the metabolism of estrogen, which is the main hormone involved in female sex. This delicate dance can be upset by an unbalanced microbiota, which can worsen menopausal symptoms.

You can encourage hormonal balance and lessen some of the discomfort related to menopause by taking care of your gut health.

3. Defense against Illness

General health depends on having a strong immune system, especially as we get older. Do you know where a good chunk of our immune system cells are located? The gut, you guessed it! Our immune system's reactions to infections, allergies, and inflammation are shaped by interactions between the microbiota and the immune system.

Our immune system is more resilient when the gut flora is healthy. On the other hand, a compromised immune system can make us more vulnerable to autoimmune diseases and infections.

4. Vitality and Energy

Are you exhausted and sluggish? Your instincts may be the key. Essential nutrients, including B vitamins and short-chain fatty acids, are produced by the microbiota. These substances provide energy to our cells, improve the synthesis of energy, and support general health.

You can regain the energy levels you believed to be lost to aging by cultivating a diversified and well-balanced gut microbiota.

The Road Ahead

This book takes us on a gut-rebooting journey designed especially for ladies over forty. We'll look at seven scientifically proven practices that can help you lose weight, boost your energy, and heal your gut microbiota. These practices include mindful eating, movement, stress reduction, hydration, intermittent fasting, and sleep optimization.

Are you prepared to discover inner glowing wellness? Let's explore the research, useful advice, and motivational tales that will enable you to recover your gut health and flourish past the age of forty.

CHAPTER ONE

The Science Underpinning Gut Health

In recent times, there has been a growing interest in the topic of gut health from researchers, medical professionals, and the general public. This recent attention is warranted because there is growing evidence that our general well-being is significantly impacted by the health of our gut. The gut affects almost every part of our physiology, from the immune system and mental health to digestion and food absorption.

We'll go into the science underlying this difficult and intriguing issue of gut health in this thorough examination, solving the puzzles of the gut microbiota, analyzing the complex relationship between the gut and the brain, and looking at the function of inflammation in gut health.

Basics of Microbiome

The gut microbiome, a huge and diverse community of bacteria that live in our gastrointestinal tract, is fundamental to gut health. The gut microbiome, which is made up of bacteria, fungi, viruses, and other microorganisms, is a dynamic and diverse community that carries out a wide range of tasks vital to human health and well-being.

The breakdown and absorption of nutrients from the food we eat is one of the main functions of the gut microbiota. Specific bacterial strains generate digestive enzymes that facilitate the body's absorption of vital nutrients and energy from complex carbs, proteins, and lipids. Furthermore, the gut microbiome supports immunological regulation, pathogen defense, and gut barrier integrity, which is an essential first line of defense against dangerous drugs and bacteria.

A multitude of factors, including genetics, diet, lifestyle, and environmental exposures, impact the composition of the gut microbiome. Although every person has a different microbiome, studies have indicated that certain patterns of microbial diversity are linked to improved health outcomes and that disruptions to the microbiome are associated with a variety of illnesses, such as diabetes, obesity, inflammatory bowel disease, and even mental health disorders.

Experts advise eating a wide variety of fiber-rich plant-based foods as well as fermented foods like yogurt, kefir, sauerkraut, and kimchi, which contain good probiotic bacteria, to maintain a healthy gut microbiota. In addition, frequent exercise, reducing stress, and abstaining from antibiotic usage can all support gut bacteria diversity and resilience.

The Gut-Brain Axis: The Impact of Your Gut on Your Mood and Vitality

The gut and the brain are connected by the gut-brain axis, a bidirectional communication network that enables them to interact and affect one another. Numerous physiological functions, such as digestion, metabolism, immunological response, mood, and cognition, are all critically regulated by this complex interaction.

The synthesis of neurotransmitters, which are chemical messengers that travel between nerve cells, is one of the main ways that the gut affects the brain. Numerous neurotransmitters, are produced in the gut and have been linked to mood regulation, stress response, and cognitive function, including serotonin, dopamine, and gamma-aminobutyric acid (GABA).

Furthermore, a range of metabolites and signaling molecules that are produced by the gut microbiota might affect behavior and brain function. For instance, certain bacterial strains have been found to generate short-chain fatty acids (SCFAs), which have been demonstrated to have anti-inflammatory properties and may offer protection against neurodegenerative illnesses such as Parkinson's and Alzheimer's.

On the other hand, the stomach's motility, the release of digesting enzymes, and the permeability of the gut barrier are all greatly influenced by the brain. Particularly stress has been demonstrated to impair gut health and change the makeup of the gut flora, resulting in symptoms including diarrhea, bloating, and abdominal pain.

It is not unexpected that changes to gut health have been linked to the emergence of mood disorders such as anxiety and depression, given the close relationship between the brain and the gut. Studies have indicated that there may be a common underlying pathophysiology between mood disorders and diseases such as irritable bowel syndrome (IBS) in people.

Disruptions to the gut-brain axis have also been connected to altered energy levels and cognitive performance, in addition to mood problems. Chronic fatigue syndrome (CFS) and fibromyalgia are illnesses marked by extreme weariness, pain, and cognitive dysfunction. Dysbiosis (imbalanced microbial composition), chronic inflammation, and gut permeability have all been linked to these conditions.

Experts advise adopting a gut-friendly diet high in fiber, fermented foods, and omega-3 fatty acids to maintain a healthy gut-brain axis and optimize mood and energy levels. They also advise practicing stress-reduction strategies like yoga, meditation, and deep breathing exercises. In addition, establishing social ties, prioritizing sleep, and engaging in regular exercise can all support a healthy gut-brain axis and enhance general well-being.

Gut Health and Inflammation

As the body's natural defense against infection and injury, inflammation is an integral and necessary component of the immune response. On the other hand, persistent or dysregulated inflammation can lead to a variety of health issues, such as autoimmune illnesses, metabolic disorders, and neurodegenerative ailments.

Chronic inflammation in the context of gut health can result from several things, such as an unbalanced microbial composition, environmental pollutants, stress, and poor food. Inflammation of the gut can weaken the gut barrier, which makes it possible for dangerous materials such as germs, poisons, and partially digested food particles to enter the bloodstream—a condition referred to as "leaky gut."

Many diseases, such as autoimmune disorders including rheumatoid arthritis, multiple sclerosis, and lupus, as well as inflammatory bowel disease (IBD), irritable bowel syndrome (IBS), celiac disease, and food allergies, have been linked to a leaky gut. Furthermore, recent studies indicate that a leaky gut may contribute to the emergence of neurodegenerative illnesses like Alzheimer's and Parkinson's as well as mood disorders like anxiety and despair.

Chronic inflammation can alter the balance of the gut microbiome, favoring the growth of pathogenic bacteria and suppressing the growth of beneficial bacteria, in addition to impairing the integrity of the gut barrier. This dysbiosis has the potential to worsen inflammation, starting a vicious cycle that accelerates the onset and development of health issues associated with the gut.

Thankfully, several methods might improve gut health and lessen inflammation. Eating a diet high in fruits, vegetables, whole grains, lean meats, and healthy fats can help reduce inflammation and encourage the repair of the digestive system. Furthermore, limiting pro-inflammatory foods such as trans fats, refined sweets, and processed meats helps ease the strain on the digestive system and promote general health.

Apart from nutrition, lifestyle elements such as effective stress reduction, consistent physical activity, and sufficient sleep are crucial for reducing inflammation and promoting intestinal well-being. While regular physical activity can help modulate the immune system and reduce systemic inflammation, mindfulness practices such as meditation, yoga, and deep breathing techniques can help lower stress levels and promote relaxation.

In essence, the area of gut health science is dynamic and varied, encompassing a wide range of linked elements such as inflammation, the gut-brain axis, and the gut microbiota. We may maximise our general well-being and discover the secret to bright health and vitality by comprehending the intricate interactions between these variables and implementing evidence-based intestinal health support techniques.

CHAPTER 2

Habit 1: Periodic Fasting for Restoring the Gut

Recent years have seen a notable increase in the use of intermittent fasting (IF) as a dietary strategy for fostering weight loss, enhancing metabolic health, and bolstering general well-being. However intermittent fasting has advantages that go far beyond just cutting calories; new studies indicate that it may also aid in gut healing and the maintenance of a balanced microbiota.

Different Techniques for Intermittent Fasting

There are various fasting regimens that fall under the umbrella of intermittent fasting, all of which alternate between eating and fasting times. Among the most popular techniques for intermittent fasting are:

1. Feeding Restricted by Time (TRF): With this approach, the daily window for eating is restricted to a set period, usually between 8 and 12 hours. For instance, a person following TRF might fast for the other fourteen hours of the day and consume all of their meals inside a 10-hour window, such as from 8 am to 6 pm.

2. ADF, or alternate-day fasting: When following an ADF, people alternate between feast days, when they eat anything they want, and fasting days when they eat very little to no calories. Fasting days can involve ingesting only

water, herbal tea, or very low-calorie foods, depending on the variety.

3. 5:2 Fasting: In this method, people eat normally five days a week and limit their consumption of calories to 500–600 on the two non-consecutive days. People usually eat one modest dinner or two snacks on fasting days to reach their daily calorie intake.

4. Extended Fasting: This type of fasting is keeping a longer period without food, usually from one to several days or even weeks. In order to maintain electrolyte balance and hydration during prolonged fasts, people only drink water or herbal tea.

Every intermittent fasting technique has its own advantages and disadvantages, so people can select the one that most closely matches their preferences, lifestyle, and health objectives.

Increased Gut Health Benefits

Numerous positive impacts on gut health have been demonstrated by intermittent fasting, many of which are mediated by modifications in the gut flora. The following are some of the main advantages of intermittent fasting for gut restoration:

1. Encourages Diversity in the Gut Microbiome: Research indicates that by causing times of feast and famine that stimulate the growth of good bacteria and prevent the spread of dangerous pathogens, intermittent fasting may support a more diversified and balanced gut microbiome.

2. Diminishes Inflammation in the Gut: Many gastrointestinal illnesses, such as irritable bowel syndrome (IBS) and inflammatory bowel disease (IBD), are characterized by chronic inflammation in the stomach. It has been demonstrated that intermittent fasting lowers gut inflammatory indicators, which may lessen inflammation-related symptoms and damage.

3. Improves Function of the Gut Barrier: By lowering oxidative stress and encouraging the creation of mucin, a protective protein that aids in preventing the entrance of hazardous substances, intermittent fasting may enhance the integrity of the gut barrier—the protective layer of cells that lines the intestinal wall.

4. Adjusts Hormones in the Gut: Gut hormones that are important in controlling hunger, metabolism, and energy balance, including

ghrelin, leptin, and peptide YY, can be secreted in response to intermittent fasting. Intermittent fasting may enhance satiety, control blood sugar, and aid in weight management by influencing these hormones.

5. Helps Promote Autophagy: In order to preserve cellular health and function, damaged or malfunctioning cellular components are recycled and eliminated through the process of autophagy. It has been demonstrated that intermittent fasting increases autophagy in the stomach and other tissues, possibly encouraging cellular regeneration and repair.

All things considered, intermittent fasting provides a comprehensive strategy for gut healing, addressing important aspects of preserving gut health and promoting general well-being.

Realistic Guidance for Execution

To guarantee success and adherence, intermittent fasting for gut regeneration must be carefully planned and considered. To get you started, consider these helpful hints:

1. Go Gradually: If you've never done intermittent fasting before, begin by progressively extending the fasting window. As your body adjusts, start with a shorter fasting window—12 hours, for example—and progressively increase it.

2. Remain Hydrated: During fasting periods, stay hydrated and promote detoxification and digestion by consuming lots of water, herbal tea, and other non-caloric beverages.

3. Listen to Your Body: Modify your fasting schedule by your body's signals of hunger and fullness. You might choose to shorten your fasting window or break your fast earlier if you're experiencing extreme weariness or hunger.

4. Emphasis on Foods High in Nutrients: To supply vital nutrients and maintain intestinal health, give priority to nutrient-dense whole meals like fruits, vegetables, lean proteins, and healthy fats while breaking your fast.

5. Show Flexibility: Keep in mind that intermittent fasting is supposed to be flexible and customized to meet your unique requirements and preferences. Don't be scared to try out several fasting regimens and make adjustments as necessary to find the one that suits you the best.

6. Monitor Your Progress: Throughout your journey of intermittent fasting, note how you're feeling emotionally, cognitively, and physically. Observe any shifts in your level of energy, mood, digestion, and general well-being, and modify your strategy accordingly.

You can use fasting to enhance gut healing and promote maximum health and energy from the inside out by heeding these helpful suggestions and sticking to your intermittent fasting schedule.

CHAPTER 3

Habit 2: Eating the Correct Foods to Nourish Your Gut

Sustaining a healthy gut flora and promoting optimal gut function requires proper nutrition. This section will discuss how to feed your gut the correct foods, such as prebiotics and probiotics, foods that are good for your gut, and methods for putting together a diet that is balanced and conducive to gut healing.

Foods Good for Your Gut

Foods that enhance digestive health, lessen inflammation, and encourage the growth of good bacteria in the gut are known as gut-friendly foods. Important nutrients that are good for the intestines include:

1. Fruits and Vegetables High in Fibre: Fibre is necessary to maintain gut motility, encourage regular bowel movements, and feed the good bacteria in the gut. Try to eat a range of fruits and vegetables that are high in fiber, such as kale, apples, broccoli, spinach, and berries.

2. Complete Grains: Because they are high in fiber, vitamins, and minerals, whole grains like quinoa, brown rice, barley, and oats are great options for supporting gut health. Instead of refined grains, which have lost most of their fiber and nutrients, choose whole grain options.

3. Grains: Because they are strong in fiber and protein, legumes like beans, lentils, and chickpeas are excellent options for enhancing digestive health and encouraging fullness. To lessen the amount of phytic acid in legumes and

increase their digestibility, make sure to soak or sprout them before cooking.

4. Fermented Food Items: Foods that have undergone fermentation are high in good probiotic bacteria, which can improve digestive health by lining the gut with beneficial microorganisms. To encourage diversity in your gut microbiota, include fermented foods such as yogurt, kefir, sauerkraut, kimchi, and kombucha regularly in your diet.

5. Healthy Fats: Rich in omega-3 fatty acids, fatty fish like salmon, mackerel, and sardines are good for your gut because they reduce inflammation. Incorporate sources of healthy fats into your diet as well, such as nuts, seeds, avocados, and olive oil, to help maintain the integrity of your intestinal barrier and supply vital nutrients.

Liver and Bone Marrow

Prebiotics are indigestible fibers that act as food for good bacteria in the stomach, encouraging their development and activity. Typical sources of prebiotics include the following:

- Inulin: Found in foods such as asparagus, Jerusalem artichokes, leeks, onions, and garlic.

-FOS: (fructooligosaccharides): Present in whole grains, bananas, and chicory root.

- Resistant starch: Present in foods such as legumes, cooked and cooled potatoes, and green bananas.

Conversely, probiotics are live bacteria that, when taken in sufficient proportions, offer health advantages. Among the places to get probiotics are:

- Yoghurt: To optimize probiotic content, use plain, unsweetened yogurt that has live, active cultures.

Kefir: A fermented dairy product that resembles yogurt but has a wider variety of probiotic strains and a thinner consistency.

- Sauerkraut: Fermented cabbage high in Lactobacillus and other probiotic microorganisms.

Consuming a diet rich in foods that are high in both probiotics and prebiotics helps support a balanced gut microbiome and encourages the best possible digestive health.

Developing a Harmonious Diet for Gut-Healing

A balanced diet that heals the gut should include foods that are good for the gut while limiting or eliminating things that could be harmful. When designing a diet for gut healing, some important guidelines to bear in mind are as follows:

1. Place a Focus on Whole, Unprocessed Foods: Give priority to complete, unprocessed foods such as vegetables, fruits, whole grains, lean meats, and healthy fats. Nutrients and fiber, which are abundant in these meals, are critical for maintaining gut health and general well-being.

2. Make Use of a Range of Colours and Textures: Incorporate as many different kinds of vibrant fruits and vegetables as possible into your diet, since they offer varying amounts of fiber and phytonutrients that promote gut health.

Add foods with different textures as well to encourage chewing and aid with digestion.

3. Restrict Processed Foods and Added Sugars: Reduce the amount of processed foods, refined grains, and added sugars you consume because these can upset the balance of your gut microbiota and cause inflammation. Rather, go for whole foods and sugar substitutes like stevia, honey, and maple syrup.

4. Moderate Consumption of Saturated Fat and Red Meat: Lean red meat sources can be included in a balanced diet, but it's crucial to eat them sparingly and choose lean cuts whenever you can. Reduce the amount of saturated fats you eat, especially processed foods, full-fat dairy products, and red meat, as they might aggravate inflammation and other digestive disorders.

5. Maintain Hydration: Maintaining intestinal motility and aiding in digestion requires adequate hydration. Along with consuming lots of water throughout the day, you should think about including foods high in water content, such as citrus fruits, cucumbers, and watermelon, in your diet.

Through adherence to these recommendations and the integration of gut-friendly items into your diet, you may construct a well-rounded and healthy eating regimen that bolsters intestinal health and fosters general well-being. To determine the food plan that is most effective for you, always pay attention to your body's signals and change as necessary.

CHAPTET 4

Habit 3: Hydration and Digestive Health

Staying hydrated is essential for preserving gut health and promoting general well-being. This section will discuss the benefits of herbal teas for supporting gut health, the significance of water for gut health, and doable methods for maintaining optimal wellness through hydration.

Water's Function in the Gut

Almost all physiological functions in the body, including digestion and food absorption, depend on water. Sustaining the health of the gastrointestinal tract and preserving normal digestive function in the context of gut health requires enough water.

Encouraging food and waste to pass through the digestive tract is one of water's main roles in the gut. Maintaining adequate water lowers the likelihood of constipation by softening feces and making it easier to pass. Water also aids in the proper absorption and utilization of vital vitamins, minerals, and other nutrients by the body by dissolving and transferring nutrients from the digestive system into the bloodstream.

Moreover, water is essential for preserving the integrity of the intestinal wall's protective layer of cells, known as the gut barrier. Maintaining adequate hydration lowers the risk of irritation, inflammation, and damage to the intestinal epithelium by keeping the mucosal lining of the gut moist and healthy. This helps to maintain healthy immune function and stops dangerous compounds from leaking into the bloodstream from the stomach, a condition called "leaky gut."

Conversely, dehydration can result in several digestive problems, such as gas, bloating, and constipation. In addition to impairing gut barrier function, chronic dehydration raises the risk of gastrointestinal conditions like irritable bowel syndrome (IBS) and inflammatory bowel disease (IBD).

Herbal Teas and Digestive Health

Herbal teas can help promote intestinal health and hydration in addition to plain water. Herbal teas are great options for supporting gut wellness because many of them contain ingredients that have been demonstrated to have anti-inflammatory, antibacterial, and digestive-supportive qualities.

The following are some of the best herbal teas for supporting the gut:

1. Tea with Peppermint: For many years, people have turned to peppermint tea as a natural cure for digestive problems like gas, bloating, and indigestion. The menthol in peppermint leaves the digestive tract's muscles relaxed, preventing spasms and encouraging more easily digested food.

2. Tea with Ginger: The anti-inflammatory and digestive-supportive qualities of ginger tea are widely recognized. It is a fantastic option for people with digestive problems like IBS because it can aid with nausea relief, better digestion, and decreased intestinal inflammation.

3. Tea with Chamomile: Tea made from chamomile is highly valued for its ability to relax and soothe the digestive system. For those with gastrointestinal problems like IBD or IBS, it's a great option because it helps ease pain and cramping, induce relaxation, and reduce inflammation.

4. Dandelion Root Tea: Packed with bitter chemicals and antioxidants, dandelion root tea promotes healthy liver function and digestion. It is a useful supplement to a gut-healing regimen since it can aid in bile production, cleansing, and good digestion.

5. Tea with Licorice Root: For ages, traditional medicine has utilized licorice root tea to alleviate gastrointestinal distress and promote intestinal well-being. It has ingredients that support the development of good bacteria in the

gut, shield the intestinal lining, and lessen inflammation.

Herbal teas can be a delightful and hydrating method to improve gut health and enhance general wellness that you can incorporate into your daily routine. Try a range of flavors and variations to determine which teas are best for your digestive system.

Hydration Is Key to Optimal Wellness

Maintaining optimal wellness and advancing general health depends on drinking enough water. The following useful tips will help you make sure you drink enough water throughout the day:

1. Make a lot of water intake: Try to consume eight 8-ounce glasses of water or more if you live in a hot region or are an active person each day. Carry a reusable water bottle with you during the day to serve as a constant reminder to stay hydrated.

2. Include Foods That Are Hydrating: Since many fruits and vegetables are high in water, they can help you stay hydrated overall. To increase your water intake, include foods high in water, such as cucumbers, watermelon, oranges, strawberries, and celery in your diet.

3. Drink Herbal Teas: Drinking herbal teas all day long can help with digestion and general well-being in addition to adding extra water. Try a range of flavors and variations to choose which teas you prefer.

4. Limit Dehydrating Beverages: As these can increase fluid loss and lead to dehydration, limit your intake of dehydrating beverages such as alcohol, caffeinated drinks, and sugary sodas.

5. Listen to Your Body: Whenever you feel thirsty, drink water by paying attention to your body's cues. Moreover, keep an eye on the color of your urine. Light yellow

Or straw-colored urine indicates that you are properly hydrated, however dark yellow or amber pee could be an indication of dehydration.

You can support optimal gut health and promote overall wellness from the inside out by making hydration a priority and including foods and herbal teas that are good for the gut in your daily routine. Always be aware of your body's needs for hydration and adapt as necessary to make sure you're getting enough fluids each day.

CHAPTER 5

Habit 4: Mindful Eating and Gut Sensitivity

Promoting optimal gut health and general well-being requires developing habits like mindful eating and gut awareness. By practicing mindfulness when making food choices, identifying triggers related to eating, and tuning into signals from the gut-brain, people can strengthen their connection with their bodies and promote digestive health.

Conscientiously Eating

The practice of mindful eating involves paying attention to the sensory components of food, paying attention to fullness and hunger signals, and bringing consciousness and intention to the eating experience. People can improve their relationship with food, aid in improved digestion, and make more deliberate decisions about what and how they eat by practicing mindful eating.

Among the fundamentals of mindful eating are:

1. **Savouring Every Bite: Give your food enough time to properly develop its flavors, textures, and scents. Chew gently and deliberately, giving yourself time to appreciate every taste.

2. No Distractions While Eating: When dining, keep electronics like computers, cellphones, and TVs to a minimum. Rather, concentrate on the eating process and the feelings of hunger, fullness, and satisfaction.

3. Paying Attention to Your Body: Eat per your body's natural signals by paying attention to your hunger and fullness signs. Observe your physical, mental, and emotional responses to various foods.

4. Practising Gratitude: Develop an attitude of thankfulness for the sustenance that comes from the food you eat. Give thanks to the farmers, producers, and other people who work so hard to get food on your table.

5. Nonjudgmental Approach: Take a nonjudgmental approach to eating, devoid of

moralizing, guilt, or shame. Embrace your dietary decisions with care and compassion, understanding that each meal presents a chance for development.

You may improve digestion, boost overall gut health, and cultivate a more pleasant and harmonious relationship with food by implementing mindful eating techniques into your daily routine.

Identifying Food Stressors

Food triggers are substances or foods that, in certain people, might make digestive symptoms worse or cause unfavourable reactions. Gluten, dairy, refined sugars, artificial additives, and highly processed meals are common food triggers.

A key component of gut awareness is understanding your unique dietary triggers and how they impact your digestion and general health. Maintaining a food journal can help you spot potential trigger foods and make educated dietary decisions by showing trends between your diet and digestive problems.

The following are some methods for identifying food triggers:

1. **Food Journaling:** Keep track of everything you consume, including food and drink, as well as any symptoms or aftereffects you encounter. To find possible trigger foods, look for trends and connections between particular foods and stomach issues.

2. **Diet of Elimination:** Remove typical trigger foods from your diet, such as dairy,

gluten, and processed foods, for a short while, and observe your body's reaction. One food at a time gradually reintroduces the others while keeping an eye out for any changes in symptoms or responses.

3. **Awareness of Symptoms:** Pay attention to how your body reacts to various foods and substances. Be mindful of symptoms such as lethargy, gas, diarrhea, constipation, bloating, and abdominal pain, as they could point to an inflammatory response to a particular food.

4. **Looking for Expert Advice:** Consider consulting a certified dietitian or another healthcare professional with expertise in digestive health if you're finding it difficult to recognize food triggers on your own. They can offer direction, encouragement, and tailored suggestions to assist you in making informed

food decisions and successfully managing digestive issues.

You may make informed dietary decisions and promote optimal gut function by learning more about your unique food triggers and how they impact your digestive health.

Brain-Gut Signals

The gut and the brain are connected by the gut-brain axis, a bidirectional communication network that enables them to interact and affect one another. Gut-brain communication is essential for controlling mood, digestion, hunger, and general health.

Paying attention to the feelings and signals that originate from the gut, such as hunger, fullness, cravings, and emotional reactions to food, is part of tuning into gut-brain communication. People can support good digestive health and gain a deeper awareness of their body's requirements by paying attention to these signals and thoughtfully responding to them.

Among the methods for focusing on gut-brain communication are:

1. Mindful Consumption: Develop mindful eating practices to increase your awareness of the sensory components of food as well as your body's signals of hunger and fullness. Before you eat, take a moment to check in with your body and determine whether you're eating for habit, boredom, or stress.

2. **Diary: ** To keep note of your eating patterns, feelings, and symptoms related to your stomach, keep a food and mood journal. To learn

more about the relationship between your gut and brain, observe any trends or connections in the way your diet, emotions, and digestive health are related.

3. **Awareness of Emotions:** Be mindful of how your emotions and stress levels impact your digestion, dietary preferences, and hunger. Utilise stress-reduction strategies like mindfulness, deep breathing, and meditation to lessen emotional eating and promote gut health.

4. **Natural Consumption:** Accept the tenets of intuitive eating, which include paying attention to your body's signals of hunger and fullness, satisfying your cravings, and putting your faith in it to make the right dietary decisions. You may promote good gut-brain communication and cultivate a more harmonious relationship with food by eating intuitively.

By practicing mindfulness when eating, identifying triggers related to food, and tuning into gut-brain signals, people can enhance their general well-being and digestive health by becoming more aware of their bodies' requirements. You can nurture your stomach from the inside out and develop a more positive, empowered connection with food by regularly putting these behaviors into practice.

CHAPTER SIX

Habit 5: Mobility and Gut Motility

In addition to being vital for maintaining general physical health, movement is also important for enhancing gut motility and digestive efficiency. This section will discuss the benefits of yoga for digestion, the significance of exercise for gut health, and methods for avoiding sedentary behavior to promote healthy gut motility.

Healthy Gut Exercise

Frequent physical activity lowers the risk of constipation, supports overall digestive function, and promotes gut motility, among many other benefits for gut health. Exercise helps to move food through the digestive system more quickly and prevents stagnation by stimulating the muscles of the digestive tract.

The following are some of the main advantages of exercise for gut health:

1. **Supports Gut Tissue:** Peristalsis, the rhythmic contractions of the digestive tract muscles that move food through the intestines, is aided by exercise. Exercise can help avoid constipation and encourage regular bowel movements by enhancing gut motility.

2. **Decreases the Chance of Digestive Problems:** A lower incidence of common digestive problems such as irritable bowel syndrome (IBS), inflammatory bowel disease (IBD), and constipation has been linked to

regular physical activity. Exercise promotes overall gut health by lowering inflammation, regulating bowel function, and more.

3. **Promotes Diversity in the Gut Microbiome:** It has been demonstrated that exercise has a beneficial impact on the diversity and composition of the gut microbiota. A more varied and balanced microbiome is linked to regular physical exercise, and this is crucial for preserving good gut health and general well-being.

4. Enhances Stress Reduction: Exercise is a highly effective way to relieve stress, and lower stress levels have been shown to have a positive effect on digestive health. Consistent stress is linked to gastrointestinal problems such as gas, discomfort in the abdomen, and altered bowel

patterns; therefore, exercising to relieve stress can be good for gut health.

Including a range of physical activities in your regimen, such as swimming, cycling, jogging, walking, and weight training, can enhance overall digestive health and encourage intestinal motility.

Yoga and Reflux

Yoga is a mind-body discipline that enhances health and well-being by combining physical postures, breathing techniques, and meditation. Yoga has many advantages for mental and emotional well-being, but it can also improve gastrointestinal and digestive processes.

Yoga can aid in digestion in several ways, including:

1. **Increases Digestive Organ Activity:** Twists, forward folds, and mild twists are a few of the yoga positions that can help activate the digestive tract's muscles and organs, enhancing gut motility and facilitating digestion.

2. **Decreases Tension:** Yoga is well renowned for its capacity to ease tension and encourage relaxation, both of which are beneficial to digestive health. Regular yoga practice can help regulate stress levels and maintain gut health because long-term stress can interfere with digestion and lead to gastrointestinal problems.

3. **Boosts the Mind-Body Link:** By fostering a closer relationship between the mind and body, yoga helps people become more perceptive of their internal signals and bodily experiences. People who engage in mindfulness

and body awareness practices are better able to identify and react to gut signals, such as those related to hunger, fullness, and discomfort during digestion.

4. Encourages Nutritious Eating Practices: Yoga helps people to pay attention to their bodies' signals of hunger and fullness and to eat mindfully. People can promote optimal digestion and have a better relationship with food by engaging in mindful eating practices.

Even a couple of times a week of yoga practice can make a big difference in your general health and digestive system. You can enhance intestinal motility and encourage good digestion by concentrating on poses that target the digestive organs, whether you practice at home or in a class.

Steer Clear of Sedentary Habits

Prolonged sitting or inactivity are examples of sedentary behavior that might negatively impact gut motility and digestive health. Long stretches of sitting can impede digestion, raise the chance of constipation, and cause gastrointestinal distress.

Take into consideration implementing the following tactics into your daily routine to prevent sedentary behavior and promote gastrointestinal motility:

1. **Take Frequent Breaks from Movement:** A short mobility break should be taken throughout the day to break up extended periods of sitting. Every hour, set a timer to remind yourself to get up, stretch, and take a little stroll.

2. Include Physical Exercise:** Make frequent exercise sessions a part of your weekly routine to prioritize physical activity. To support intestinal motility and general health, try to get in at least 30 minutes of moderate-intensity exercise most days of the week.

3. **Use a Standing Desk:** To enable you to switch between sitting and standing during the day, think about utilizing an adjustable workstation or standing desk. Standing desks can promote greater movement and activity while assisting in lowering the amount of time spent sitting.

4. **Take the Stairs:** Whenever feasible, choose the stairs over the lift. One easy and efficient strategy to increase your daily physical activity and improve your gastrointestinal motility is to climb stairs.

5. Take Up Active Interests: Look for pastimes and pursuits that require movement and physical exertion, such as sports, dancing, hiking, or gardening. Taking part in pleasant physical activities can promote overall well-being and intestinal health.

By abstaining from inactive lifestyle choices and integrating consistent physical exercise into your everyday regimen, you may enhance digestion, boost gastrointestinal motility, and elevate your general health. Making movement a priority is crucial for maintaining optimal gut health, whether that is achieved through exercise, yoga, or just staying active all day long.

CHAPTER 7

Habit 6: Gut Harmony and Stress Management

A vital component of preserving gut health and general well-being is stress management. Prolonged stress can have a significant impact on the stomach, impairing digestion, changing the makeup of the gut flora, and aggravating gastrointestinal complaints. This part will discuss how stress affects gut health, how to relax to support gut harmony, and how important it is to prioritize taking care of oneself for the best possible health.

The Effect of Stress on Gut Health

The gut-brain axis is a complicated network that connects the gut and brain in an intricate way. The enteric nervous system (ENS), which regulates the operation of the gastrointestinal tract, and the central nervous system (CNS) can communicate continuously because of this bidirectional communication mechanism.

The body's stress response system is triggered by stress, either physical or psychological since the brain interprets stress as a threat. Stress chemicals like cortisol and adrenaline are released as a result, and these can have a significant impact on gut health. These impacts include:

1. Modified Digestive Process: Constipation, diarrhea, bloating, and abdominal discomfort are just a few of the symptoms that can arise from chronic stress's disruption of the digestive system. Stress hormones have the power to slow down digestion, alter how the gastrointestinal muscles contract, and increase the permeability of the gut, which allows dangerous compounds to seep into the circulation.

2. Unbalanced Microbiota in the Gut: The community of microbes that live in the gastrointestinal system, known as the gut microbiota, can change in composition and diversity as a result of stress. Functional dyspepsia, inflammatory bowel disease (IBD), and irritable bowel syndrome (IBS) have all been linked to changes in the makeup of the gut microbiota.

3. **Inflamed Body Parts:** Prolonged stress can cause intestinal inflammation, which can result in immunological dysregulation and tissue damage. Gut inflammation that persists over time has been connected to the emergence of gastrointestinal illnesses and other systemic health issues.

All things considered, long-term stress can be harmful to gut health, impairing general well-being and accelerating the onset or aggravation of digestive diseases.

Meditation Methods

By using relaxation techniques, gut harmony can be promoted and the negative effects of stress on gut health can be lessened. By triggering the body's relaxation response, these methods seek to counteract the physiological effects of stress and encourage a calm, balanced state of mind.

Here are a few successful relaxation methods for reducing stress and promoting intestinal health:

1.   **Deep Breathing Exercises**: Diaphragmatic breathing and belly breathing are two examples of deep breathing techniques that can assist trigger the body's relaxation response and lower stress levels. Spend a few minutes everyday deep breathing exercises to help you relax and clear your head.

2. **Muscle relaxation with progressive muscles:** To relieve physical stress and encourage relaxation, PMR entails methodically tensing and relaxing various muscle groups in the body. Regularly engage in PMR exercises to

ease tense muscles and symptoms associated with stress.

3. **Meditation with mindfulness:** Practicing mindfulness meditation entails bringing attention to the here and now while letting go of judgment and allowing ideas and feelings to flow and go. Frequent mindfulness meditation practice can enhance general well-being, support emotional balance, and lower stress.

4. Tai Chi and Yoga: Mind-body exercises like yoga and tai chi combine breathing exercises, meditation, and moderate movement to help people unwind and reduce stress. These exercises can lower stress levels, support gastrointestinal health, and enhance mental clarity, flexibility, and balance.

5. [Directed Visual Aids:] Using guided imagery, one can visualize serene and relaxing situations or memories to promote relaxation and well-being. Regularly engage in guided imagery activities to lower stress and foster inner calm.

Putting Self-Care First

Setting aside time for self-care is crucial for fostering gut harmony and stress management in addition to relaxing methods. Self-care entails making conscious decisions to support your mental, emotional, and physical health as well as to lower your stress level and build resilience.

The following are some self-care techniques that promote gut health and general well-being:

1. Eating Healthily: Give top priority to wholesome, entire foods including fruits,

vegetables, whole grains, lean meats, and healthy fats that promote intestinal health. Processed foods, sugary snacks, and items that can worsen digestive symptoms should be avoided or limited.

2. **Regular Exercise**: Exercise on a regular basis to enhance general health and wellbeing, lower stress levels, and encourage digestive motility. Make fitness a regular habit by finding things you enjoy doing and incorporating them into your daily schedule.

3. Getting Enough Sleep: Make it a priority to obtain adequate restorative sleep every night in order to promote gut health and stress reduction. To encourage restful sleep, aim for 7-9 hours of high-quality sleep each night and adopt healthy sleep hygiene practices.

4. **Social Connection:** To offer social support and lessen feelings of loneliness and isolation, cultivate ties with friends, family, and loved ones. Make time to engage in meaningful social interactions and prioritize face-to-face or virtual connections with people.

5. **Mindfulness Practices:** To increase self-awareness, lower stress levels, and build resilience, incorporate mindfulness exercises into your daily routine, such as journaling, meditation, or nature walks.

6. **Determining Limits: ** To safeguard your time, energy, and well-being, clearly define boundaries with regard to work, relationships, and duties. Prioritise the things that make you happy and fulfilled and learn to say no to obligations or activities that deplete your energy.

Making self-care a priority and including relaxing methods in your daily routine will help you manage stress, maintain gut harmony, and advance your general health and well-being. Recall that taking care of oneself is not selfish; rather, it is necessary to preserve resilience, equilibrium, and vitality in the fast-paced world of today.

CHAPTER 8

Habit 7: Sleep and Gut Healing

Sleep is essential for gut health and healing as well as general health and well-being. This section will discuss the significance of sleep for gut healing, how to create a good sleep schedule, and how to maintain gut health at night.

The Function of Sleep in Gut Healing

The body's natural regeneration and repair mechanisms, which include those that maintain gut health, depend on getting enough sleep. The physiological changes that occur in the body during sleep support immune response, tissue repair, and metabolic control—all of which are essential for preserving gut health.

1. Integrity of the gut barrier: The gut barrier, which is a layer of cells lining the gastrointestinal tract, needs to remain intact in order to function properly. Chronic sleep deprivation has been linked to heightened gut permeability, which makes it possible for

dangerous chemicals to enter the circulation and cause intestinal inflammation.

2. **Balance of the Gut Microbiome: ** The balance of the gut microbiome, or the community of bacteria that live in the gastrointestinal system, is mostly regulated by sleep. Sleep disturbances can change the diversity and makeup of the gut microbiota, which can result in dysbiosis, microbial imbalance, and related health issues.

3. **Control of Inflammation: ** Sleep aids in the regulation of the body's inflammatory processes, particularly gastrointestinal ones. Systemic inflammation, which has been connected to several digestive illnesses, including inflammatory bowel disease (IBD), irritable bowel syndrome (IBS), and

gastroesophageal reflux disease (GERD), is a result of chronic sleep deprivation.

4. The Digestive System: Bile acid secretion, intestinal motility, and gastric emptying are among the digestive processes that are impacted by sleep. These functions can be hampered by sleep patterns, which can result in symptoms of the digestive system such as gas, indigestion, and bloating.

All things considered, getting enough sleep is critical to promoting gut healing and preserving ideal gut health. Making getting enough sleep a priority can guard against stomach issues and improve general health.

Creating Sleep-Healthy Routines

Sleep hygiene, or creating healthy sleep habits, is crucial to getting a restorative and peaceful sleep. The following are some methods to enhance the quality of your sleep and encourage gut healing:

1. **Maintain a Regular Sleep Schedule: ** Every day, including on the weekends, go to bed and wake up at the same time. Maintaining consistency improves the quality of your sleep and aids your body's internal clock.

2. Establish a Calm Bedtime Schedule: Create a relaxing nighttime ritual to let your body know when it's time to relax. Your body and mind can be ready for sleep with the aid of activities like reading, having a warm bath, deep breathing exercises, meditation, or relaxing music.

3. **Establish a Cosy Sleep Environment: ** Make sure your bedroom is quiet, dark, and cold so that you can sleep well. Invest in pillows and mattresses that are comfortable for you, and get rid of any distractions that could keep you from sleeping, such as electronics and loud noises.

4. Restrict Electronics and Stimulants Before Bed: In the hours before going to bed, stay away from nicotine, caffeine, and stimulating activities (including strenuous exercise or screen time). Electronic device blue light can inhibit melatonin production and disrupt sleep, thus it's advisable to avoid screens at least one hour before bed.

5. Be Aware of Your Diet: Before going to bed, stay away from large meals, spicy foods, and liquids in excess as these can make you uncomfortable and interfere with your sleep. If

you're hungry right before bed, choose lighter, easier-to-digest snacks; stay away from coffee and alcohol, as these can disrupt your sleep.

6. **Control Tension:** Anxiety and stress can aggravate stomach issues and impair sleep. To help you relax and de-stress before bed, try stress-reduction methods like progressive muscle relaxation, journaling, or mindfulness meditation.

You may create healthy sleep habits and aid in gut healing by implementing these techniques into your evening routine.

Gut Support at Night

Although sleep is necessary for gut healing, you can additionally take the following particular steps to promote your gut health while you sleep:

First, prebiotics and probiotics: To maintain gut microbiota balance, think about taking a probiotic supplement or eating foods high in probiotics, such as yogurt, kefir, and fermented vegetables. Foods high in prebiotics, such as bananas, oats, onions, and garlic, can also support gut health by nourishing good gut bacteria.

2. **Enzymes for Digestion:** Before going to bed, some people find that taking digestive enzyme supplements supports healthy digestion and eases discomfort related to digesting at night. By aiding in the more effective breakdown of meals, digestive enzymes can lower the chance of bloating, gas, and indigestion.

3. Herbal Treatments: During the night, gut health can be supported by some herbal teas and supplements that have soothing and digestive-supportive qualities. Popular choices that support relaxation and aid in calming the digestive system before bed are chamomile, ginger, and peppermint teas.

4. **Surfactant:** Staying hydrated is important during the day, but pay attention to how much fluid you consume right before bed to prevent frequent urine from keeping you awake. Before going to bed, you can improve digestion and encourage relaxation by consuming a modest amount of water or herbal tea without filling up your bladder.

5. **Gentle Movement:** Stretching or gentle movement before bed can help release tension in the muscles and calm the body, which may

improve digestion and the quality of sleep. To assist your body in getting ready for sleep, think about adding stretches or light yoga into your nightly routine.

You can enhance your sleeping environment and encourage gut healing while you sleep by including these nocturnal gut support techniques in your routine.

Maintaining optimal gut health and promoting gut healing requires making sleep a priority and developing appropriate sleep habits. You may support digestive wellness and general well-being by making getting enough sleep a priority, adhering to proper sleep hygiene, and using nightly gut support techniques.

Keep in mind that getting enough sleep is essential for maintaining good health and that, for the best possible gut healing and general well-being, it should be prioritized along with diet, exercise, and stress reduction.

CHAPTER 9

Habit 8:Self-Care Practices

Self-care is not an extravagance; rather, it is essential for gut health and general wellness. We'll go into how important it is to prioritize self-care, daily self-care routines for gut regeneration, and developing a positive outlook for long-term success in this section.

Putting Self-Care First for General Wellness

Whatever intentional action is done to maintain or enhance one's physical, mental, emotional, and spiritual well-being is referred to as self-care. Making self-care a priority is essential for preserving equilibrium, lowering stress levels, and fostering general wellness, which includes gut health.

1. **Reduction of Stress:** Prolonged stress can negatively impact gut health by affecting gut barrier function, gut microbial balance, and digestion. Stress on the gut can be lessened by making self-care activities that encourage relaxation and stress reduction a priority. Examples of these activities include deep

breathing exercises, meditation, and time spent in nature.

2. **Emotional Well-Being:** Since emotions can affect gut function and vice versa, emotional well-being and gut health are intimately related. Self-care activities that boost mental well-being, including journaling, counseling, or quality time with loved ones, can enhance general wellness and aid in gut healing.

3. **Healthy Habits: ** Practicing self-care entails forming wholesome lifestyle choices that promote general well-being, such as consistent exercise, enough sleep, and a well-balanced diet. Making these routines a priority can improve gut health and add to a feeling of vitality and well-being.

4. Limitations and Introspective Compassion: Two crucial components of self-care are establishing boundaries and engaging in self-compassion exercises. Saying no to commitments that take up your energy and engaging in self-compassion during trying times can help safeguard your mental and emotional health, build resilience, and support gut health.

Making self-care a priority helps people develop resilience, lower their stress levels, and support their general wellness, which includes gut health.

Regular Self-Care Activities for Restoring Gut Health

Including regular self-care activities in your routine can help with gut healing and enhance general well-being. The following self-care techniques are specially designed to promote intestinal health:

1. Mindful Consumption: To eat mindfully, one must become aware of the sensory aspects of the process, as well as the signals of hunger and fullness, as well as the physiological effects of various foods. You may promote gut health and optimal digestion by eating thoughtfully.

2. **Aqueous:** Because water promotes healthy digestion, nutritional absorption, and the passage of waste products through the digestive tract, maintaining adequate hydration is crucial for gut health. Develop the practice of drinking a lot of water all day long to aid in gut healing and general well-being.

3. **Gut-Supportive Nutrition:** By feeding good gut bacteria and encouraging regular bowel

movements, a diet high in fiber, fruits, vegetables, and fermented foods can promote gut health. Make foods that are good for your gut a priority in your diet to help with gut healing and general health.

4. **Stress Reduction:** Stress management is essential for gut health since long-term stress can worsen symptoms associated with the gut and interfere with digestion. To support gut healing and general wellness, incorporate stress-relieving activities into your daily routine, such as meditation, deep breathing exercises, or time spent in nature.

5. Proper Sleeping Habits: Make maintaining proper sleep hygiene a top priority to aid with gut healing and general well-being. To encourage restful sleep and support gut health, aim for seven to nine hours of quality sleep per

night, create a calming bedtime routine, and stick to a regular sleep schedule.

These everyday self-care routines can help restore your gut and encourage general wellness by starting from the inside out.

Developing an Upbeat Attitude for Prolonged Achievement

Maintaining gut health and general wellness over the long run requires developing a positive outlook. A positive outlook can enhance behavior, resilience, and general well-being, which can lead to greater health and a higher standard of living.

1. **Practice Gratitude:** By focusing on what you have instead of what you need, practicing thankfulness can help you feel abundant and

well-being. To help you maintain a good outlook and advance your general well-being, set aside some time each day to think about the things you have to be thankful for, no matter how small.

2. **Filipinness and Hope:** Resilience and optimism are traits that can make overcoming obstacles easier and more graceful. To enhance your general well-being, put more emphasis on finding answers than wallowing in issues. You can also practice self-compassion and self-care at trying moments.

3. **Gracious Confirmations:** Positive affirmations are declarations that support your best traits or self-beliefs. Reframing negative thought patterns and cultivating a more positive mindset via the daily practice of positive affirmations can support gut repair and general wellness.

4. **Presence and Mindfulness:** Being mindful entails bringing consciousness to the here and now with acceptance, curiosity, and openness. You can develop a stronger sense of presence, lessen stress, and support gut health as well as general well-being by engaging in mindfulness practices.

5. **Grace for Oneself:** Treating oneself with love, understanding, and acceptance—especially while facing challenges or adversity—is an important part of practicing self-compassion. You can overcome obstacles with more resiliency and promote both gut healing and general well-being by practicing self-compassion.

You may encourage long-term success in preserving gut health and general fitness by developing an optimistic outlook. You may support gut healing and promote general well-being from the inside out by making self-care a priority, including self-care activities in your daily routine, and developing an optimistic outlook. Recall that taking care of oneself is not selfish; rather, it is necessary to preserve resilience, vitality, and balance in the fast-paced world of today.

CHAPTER 10

Combining Everything: Your Action Plan for a Gut Reboot

Having explored a range of behaviors and routines that promote gut health and general well-being, it's now time to design a customized Gut Reboot Action Plan. This plan will assist you in tracking your progress, celebrating your victories along the road, and incorporating the concepts covered throughout this book into your everyday life.

Developing Your Own Customised Programme for Gut Health

1. **Evaluate Your Present Routines:** Begin by evaluating your present lifestyle practices

about food, physical activity, rest, handling stress, and taking care of yourself. Determine what areas you can strengthen for general wellness and gut health.

2. **Set Specific Goals:** Create attainable goals for enhancing gut health based on the results of your examination. Setting specific goals will help direct your action plan, whether it's increasing the amount of gut-friendly items in your diet, starting a regular exercise regimen, or giving stress-relieving activities a top priority.

3. **Build Your Action Plan:** Divide your objectives into manageable tasks and make a thorough action plan to include them in your everyday schedule. Think about adopting the routines and behaviors that are covered in this book, like stress reduction methods, mindful

eating, consistent exercise, and self-care routines.

4. **Create Daily Routines:** To establish a customized gut wellness routine, including the habits and practices that you have selected for your everyday routine. Make time for self-care, exercise, mindful eating, and relaxation a daily priority, and set aside specific times for each of these activities.

5. **Remain Adaptable:** As you carry out your gut health regimen, be flexible and adaptive. You may face unforeseen obstacles in life, but you can continue to put your general well-being and gut health first by remaining adaptable and making changes as needed.

6. **Ask for Help:** Once you start your gut reboot journey, don't be afraid to ask friends,

family, or medical experts for support. Be in the company of individuals who will support your objectives and who can offer you support, accountability, and direction as you go.

Monitoring Development and Honouring Achievements

1. **Keep a Journal:** Record your experiences and monitor your development in a journal while you go through your gut reset. When you follow your gut wellness regimen, take note of any changes in your overall well-being, energy levels, mood, and symptoms.

2. Make Use of a Habit Monitor: To keep an eye on your daily routine and make progress towards your objectives, use an app or habit tracker. You can stay accountable and spot patterns or places

where you might need to make changes by keeping track of your behaviors.

3. **Celebrate minor Wins:** Acknowledge and celebrate all of your minor victories along the journey. Take some time to recognize and appreciate your accomplishments, whether they include eating more veggies, exercising consistently for a week, or engaging in daily mindfulness exercises.

Assess and Modify: Make sure your goals are still in line with your requirements and priorities by reviewing your progress regularly. Be prepared to modify your action plan as necessary in light of your experiences and your body's reaction.

5. Employ Self-Compassion Techniques: Throughout your gut reset journey, treat yourself

with kindness and cultivate self-compassion, particularly in the face of adversity. Recall that obstacles are a normal part of the process and that progress is not always linear. You should navigate your journey to wellness with compassion, tolerance, and kindness towards yourself.

You may nurture optimal gut health and overall wellness by making a personalized action plan for your gut reboot, monitoring your progress, and acknowledging your accomplishments along the journey. Keep in mind that every person's experience with a gut reboot is different and that by putting your health and well-being first, you're making an investment in a happier, healthier future.

CHAPTER 11

Gut Health Recipes

Including meals that are good for your stomach is a tasty and practical approach to promoting digestive health and general well-being. We'll look at a range of recipes in this part that support gut health, feed the microbiome, and offer tasty options for every meal and snack.

Smoothies to Heal the Gut

Smoothies are a great method to combine several components that help repair the gut into a tasty and portable beverage. You should try a few of these dishes:

1. **Green Smoothie for Gut-Healing:**

Ingredients: - 1/2 cup sliced cucumber; - 1 cup spinach or kale

- 1/2 cup chopped pineapple

- Half a ripe avocado

One-third cup of chia seeds

- One cup of almond milk or coconut water

- Guidelines:

1. Fill a blender with all the ingredients.

2. Blend until creamy and smooth.

3. Transfer to a glass and start sipping right away.

2. **Gut-Healing Smoothie with Berry Bliss:**

- Components:

  - A half cup of mixed berries, including raspberries, blueberries, and strawberries

  - One half banana

  - One-half cup Greek yogurt, plain

  - One tablespoon of maple syrup or honey

  -Almond milk or coconut water, half a cup

  - One spoonful of flaxseed powder

- Guidelines:

  1. Fill a blender with all the ingredients.

  2. Blend until creamy and smooth.

3. Transfer into a glass and savor the revitalizing and filling pleasure.

Gut-Nourishing Meals**

You may maintain digestive health and get critical nutrients by including foods that are good for your gut. Here are some suggestions for meals to think about:

1. **Vegetable Buddha Bowl with Quinoa:**

- Ingredients: - One cup of cooked quinoa - A variety of roasted veggies, including bell peppers, sweet potatoes, broccoli, and carrots

- Half a cup of washed and drained chickpeas

- Half a spoonful of hummus

- Fresh herbs, such as parsley or cilantro

- Lemon-tahini dressing (olive oil, garlic, lemon juice, and tahini)

- Guidelines:

1. Fill a bowl with the cooked quinoa and the roasted veggies.

2. Add hummus, fresh herbs, and chickpeas on top.

3. Add a lemon-tahini dressing drizzle.

4. Serve right now, and savor a filling and nutritious dinner.

2. Stir-fried asparagus and salmon:

Ingredients: - 1 bunch of asparagus, trimmed and chopped into bite-sized pieces; - 2 salmon fillets

- One sliced bell pepper

- One tablespoon of olive oil

- Two minced garlic cloves

- Two tablespoons tamari or soy sauce

- One tablespoon of maple syrup or honey

- Prepared cooked quinoa or brown rice for serving.

- Guidelines:

1. In a big skillet over medium heat, warm up the olive oil.

2. Add the minced garlic and heat it until fragrant, one to two minutes.

3. Place the salmon fillets in the skillet and cook them through, 3 to 4 minutes on each side.

4. Take out the fish and place it aside from the skillet.

5. Add the bell pepper and asparagus to the same skillet.

6. Stir-fry the vegetables for 4–5 minutes, or until they are crisp-tender.

7. Transfer the cooked fish back to the skillet.

8. Combine the honey and soy sauce in a small bowl.

9. Drizzle the fish and veggies with sauce.

10. Continue to stir-fry for a further one to two minutes, or until everything is well cooked and covered in sauce.

11. Toss with cooked brown rice or quinoa and serve for a tasty and wholesome supper.

Recespite-Friendly Foods

In between meals, healthy snacks can help sustain energy levels and prevent hunger. Here are some options for stomach-friendly snacks:

1. **Croatian Yoghurt Bowl:**

   Ingredients: - Greek yogurt, plain

   - Berries that are fresh, like raspberries, blueberries, or strawberries

   Nuts or granola

   - Optional: honey or maple syrup

  - Guidelines:

   1. In a small bowl or glass, arrange Greek yogurt, fresh berries, and granola or almonds.

2. If preferred, drizzle with honey or maple syrup for extra sweetness.

3. Savour as a filling and high-nutrient snack.

2. **Concoction Made at Home:**

Ingredients: - A variety of nuts, including cashews, walnuts, and almonds

- Dried fruit, including cranberries, raisins, and apricots

- Chips made of dark chocolate or cacao nibs

- Flakes of coconut

- Guidelines:

1. In a bowl, combine the almonds, coconut flakes, dark chocolate chips, and dried fruit.

2. Divide into discrete snack packs or containers to facilitate convenient on-the-go snacking.

3. Savour as a filling and convenient snack choice.

Including dishes that are good for your gut can supplement your diet with vital nutrients, aid with digestive issues, and enhance your general health. These recipes provide delectable options to support your gut health journey, whether you're having a full dinner, a pleasant snack, or a nutritious smoothie.

In Summary

Beyond Forty and Radiantly Well

We are on an important journey towards radiant wellness beyond 40, where we can embrace gut reboot practices for long-term health. We have examined the transforming potential of supporting our gut health and adopting behaviors that promote general well-being throughout this book. We have set out on a path of self-discovery and empowerment, from realizing the significance of gut health for women over 40 to delving into doable tactics for gut regeneration.

**Adopting Gut Reboot Routines for Long-Term Health

Our entire well-being is based on our gut health, which affects everything from mood and energy levels to immune system performance and digestion. We take proactive measures to nourish our bodies and cultivate radiant wellness long into our 40s and beyond by adopting gut reboot practices.

A few of the practices we have investigated on our journey include intermittent fasting, eating the correct meals for our bodies, drinking plenty of water, and placing a high priority on self-care. These practices enhance longevity, vigor, and resilience in addition to gut health. By establishing these routines in our daily lives, we create the foundation for long-term health and well-being.

Inspiring Tales of Metamorphosis

In addition to scientific insights and useful practices, we have drawn inspiration from the transformational stories of women who have taken on their gut health journeys. These tales serve as a reminder that everything is possible and that we can overcome challenges and attain radiant wellness at any age by putting our health and well-being first.

These inspiring tales highlight the importance of resiliency, willpower, and self-care as they overcome everything from digestive problems to regaining energy and vitality. They act as rays of inspiration and hope, demonstrating to us that we can change our lives and prosper in every way if we put in the necessary effort and support.

Let us take the lessons learned and embrace the road towards radiant wellness beyond 40 as we consider the ideas, tactics, and anecdotes presented in this book. As we prioritize our health, we open the door to a life full of vitality, joy, and fulfillment. Let us nourish our bodies, minds, and spirits with love, compassion, and intention.

To sum up, may we keep believing in the potential of gut health, develop lifestyle-promoting habits, and encourage others to set off on their own paths to radiant wellness over the age of forty. By working together, we can make a world in which all women, regardless of age or stage in life, have the information, resources, and confidence to lead the healthiest, happiest lives possible.